H   elp

❧ **GERRY HARRINGTON** ❧

Leabharlanna P...

Dublin...

D1439895

How Horses Help
Breaking the Barriers of Disability with Equine Assisted Therapy
© Gerry Harrington
ISBN 978-1-909116-45-0

Published in 2015 by SRA Books

Printed in the UK by TJ International, Padstow

ঙ Acknowledgements ও

First and foremost, I would like a huge thank you to go to my family and friends, who have assisted me in all my endeavours for the last fifty or so years of my life.

Special thanks to my three photographic models who helped with the images in the book, and of course, a big thank you to all those brilliant horses who put up with us on a daily basis, and have shared our confidences and experiences in their lives. Without them this book would not have been written.

I would also like to thank the students, parents, friends and colleagues of the Fortune Centre of Riding Therapy, who have provided me with so many learning experiences and practical help during my time there.

Last but not least, I am grateful to Sarah Williams and Sue Richardson, and all their staff for their help and support in the writing and publishing of this book.

This book is written in memory of Yvonne Nelson and Jennie Baillie, the founders of the Fortune Centre of Riding Therapy.

❧ Contents ❧

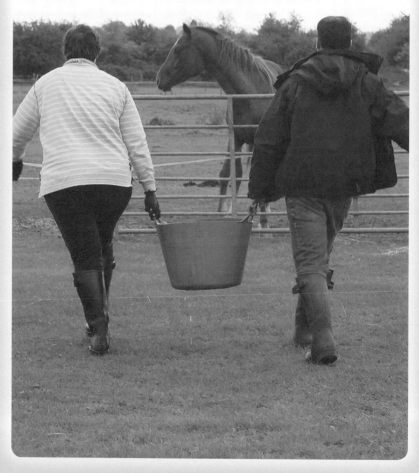

Horses and people: learning from each other.

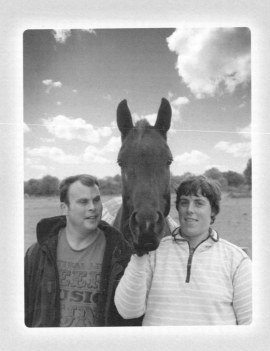

❧ Introduction ❧

Introduction

Imagine a boy. We'll call him Bill. He may look a little like your son, your cousin, your brother. Bill finds learning a challenge. His brain isn't wired like that of other people, and he doesn't always pick up on the social signals that tell the rest of us what constitutes appropriate behaviour. But Bill is energetic and cheerful, and adores being the centre of attention. He shouts and claps his hands to make sure that no one overlooks him.

Now put Bill in care of a horse. Bill loves the soft nuzzling of the horse, focused only on him. Bill soon learns that if he shouts and claps, he spooks the horse and it runs away from him. To keep the horse calm and close to him, he has to learn to be calm and quiet himself.

This is what Equine Assisted Therapy (EAT) is all about: rather than being forced to behave in often incomprehensible ways as instructed by other people, working with a horse leads a person to change their own behaviour, in order to receive the extraordinary reward of the horse's trust and affection.

There are all sorts of disorders and conditions that can be helped using EAT. For example, there are those with learning difficulties, such as Bill; some with spinal problems; others with congenital problems, such as cystic fibrosis, or chromosomal disorders such as Fragile X syndrome, Turner's syndrome or Down's syndrome. Many conditions come with other problems as the child grows, such as challenging behaviour, poor speech and lack of communication, or the absence of any social interaction skills. For instance, in autistic spectrum disorders, there are those who are hyperactive or oppositional, who tend to be very self-absorbed.

There are many other problems that may be helped by contact with a horse, such as depression, addiction and eating disorders. Some young offenders have been found to have changed their lives around following Equine Assisted Therapy.

Horses used to work, pulling ploughs or carriages, or carrying soldiers, but now we have found another, even more special job for them: they can provide more meaning to peoples' lives by just allowing them to enjoy their company, by learning how to communicate with them and care for them.

The benefits are often astounding as the horse becomes a teacher, therapist and friend.

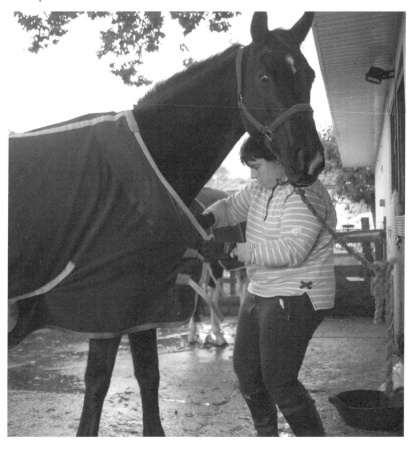

Taking care of the horse enables students to take care of themselves.

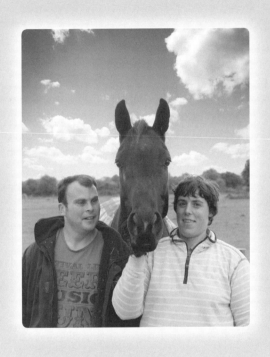

❧ Part one: ❧
Equine Assisted Therapy, what, why and how

What is Equine Assisted Therapy?

Equine Assisted Therapy (EAT). Let's start with the first word. 'Equine' means anything to do with a horse; of, or like a horse; or just horse; and derives from *equus*, the Latin for horse. The term 'assisted' means help; be present. So the horse helps the therapy. 'Therapy', or 'therapeutic' is the term for curative treatment; remedying or tending to something.

Let's go one further in stating that EAT is horses' help for gaining health. So what is 'health'? According to my dictionary, it is the soundness of body or mind. I would say that it is the well-being of body or mind. For instance, a healthy attitude is one which incorporates good, nutritious food, a certain amount of exercise, to ensure the whole body maintains a good level of fitness, and good sleeping patterns. To ensure a healthy mind, we need to consider a safe environment, good relationships, social activities, mental and emotional happiness, and choices for work and leisure, in order for us to be in a state of being well.

Therefore, EAT can be defined as: working with horses to help an individual to gain and maintain a healthy lifestyle.

Equine Assisted Therapy is an alternative way of providing different paths through peoples' lives by using the 'hook' of the horse as a special motivator.

When we are young we learn to do most things through play, and if we can retain the fun element in the learning process of our children they will continue to learn. Look at how many people love football, and so learn the basics of teamwork and the focus needed to score a goal. Most people enjoy listening to music: music can be calming and inspiring, or be danced to with a group of friends. This teaches us to be in touch with our bodies and our minds, and when dancing, can teach us to move our bodies in a rhythm that is sociable and pleasurable.

Animals, too, can help us learn. Some people may be a little nervous initially, or intimidated by larger animals, or have preconceptions about how some animals may be aggressive, but dealing with nerves and preconceptions is part of the learning process. A large football ground with many fans can also be intimidating at first, but the child who loves football will learn to overcome this.

As children, we love the feel of fur and fluffy animals, and seeing them play with each other; we like the way they come to us for attention and stroking; we like to feed them and to see a reaction when they want more; we love seeing them as young animals next to their mothers, being protected, just as we feel with our own parents; we love watching them move, and there is nothing more beautiful than seeing an elephant lumbering across the plains, a giraffe stretching up to eat the tops of trees, or a little foal cantering across the field to find his mother. We use almost all our senses in this emotional response. EAT has this fundamental human response to animals at its core.

Animals can help us learn, they can help us to make friends, and can help us to face our challenges, and make new paths and choices in our lives.

Horses, in particular, are able to help us on so many levels. For those who have never touched a horse this may be difficult to relate to at first. When caring for dogs it is essential to make sure they are fed, kept clean, exercised regularly and have a certain amount of time to play … While doing this we are learning to measure feeds, finding the right food for the dog or child, and making sure it is eating, house-trained, taking them for walks, and playing with them as much as possible. All of this constitutes basic training for the puppy.

Now take that to a much larger scale, which is what is required with a horse. Feeding does not just mean grass for most horses. Keeping them clean is an arduous job, but very satisfying, and exercise and play can heighten all our own emotions and senses.

Further on in the book, I will explain how this may help you with a young person with a 'condition'. Some conditions may be minor, but others may involve huge challenges. Students may be faced with

Asperger's syndrome or autistic spectrum disorders, deafness or blindness, Down's syndrome or Turner's syndrome, cystic fibrosis or diabetes, to name but a few. Many may have moderate learning difficulties to severe disabilities, and this can take its toll on the carer or parent. I have called them 'conditions', not because I take them lightly, but only because there are so many differing illnesses, disorders or syndromes, which are frequently associated with other difficulties.

For instance, one young girl had been born with heart problems and throughout her young life had spent months at a time in hospital undergoing various surgical operations, which prevented her from going to school and making friends. As she passed through her teenage years, she became frustrated and depressed because she was unable to keep up with her schoolwork and had difficulty keeping any new friends, which caused her to have certain behavioural problems. This turned into a spiral as she then did not want to learn and could not maintain any friendships or relationships. As she had missed so much schooling she was unable to communicate effectively with her teachers, her peers or her parents. In addition, she was of short stature and had been bullied by many of her classmates.

So, although she had been born with a physical condition, she then developed learning and behavioural problems. This is where having an individual work with horses can be so effective – it's not just one facet of that person which is called into play – every part of them is involved, challenged and changed.

EAT is particularly effective in helping students transfer skills learned when working with the horse to other situations, increasing their ability to live independently. Skills can be transferred through repetition and the continuous encouragement of a good therapist, who is able to relate the skill learnt from working with the horse to the student's own care plan needs. The therapist needs to be able to recognise the skill learnt from the horse and to use this immediately to help the student. For example, by helping a student to learn how to clean horse's clothing, they are able to emphasise the reasons why this is important, and also to highlight the importance of the student keeping their own clothing clean. They can then help the student learn how to use a washing machine for horse wear, which would, in turn, be communicated to the carer helping the student in a domestic situation, to teach the student how to use a washing machine for their own clothing.

Who would benefit?

The easy answer to this is anyone who has a basic liking of animals. Most people will benefit from some form of contact with a horse but those who will gain most are those who find the contact rewarding and pleasurable. Here we are talking mainly about people with disabilities gaining the most benefits from EAT but, as all those who work with horses know, each of us can gain pleasure and comfort simply from being near them.

The range of cognitive, psychological and physical challenges which can be addressed and managed using EAT is almost infinite. In Part two we cover just a few specific instances, but the list is far from definitive – wherever there is a human being with difficulties, there is sure to be a way that EAT can help.

The way horses help is by working on all of the difficulties a person may have, to provide a better life for that person. This holistic therapy, when working with horses, is called Equine Assisted Therapy (EAT) in the UK, although in other countries or establishments it may have a slightly different name.

Equine assisted therapy is a natural healing process that has no side effects, where the horse is the key to the motivation for healthy progression. It involves three distinct aspects – cognitive, physical and psychological – which are all interlinked.

When a young person is referred they are assessed for ability, in order to provide an individual goal/care plan. The person naturally and gradually forms a relationship with the horses and this then provides the power for continuous therapy and education.

For many young people over school age working with horses is often a dream job. During EAT, young people with special needs are taught everyday routines for the care and needs of the horses they love. They learn how to lead a horse quietly and calmly, how to groom it, how to feed it and how to keep safe when managing and working with the animal. They learn to ride with a qualified instructor/therapist and mix with like-minded peers, while learning about the social aspects of the horse in a herd, and are able to communicate with the horse without words when riding.

Horses are very sensitive to people's emotions and body language, and can enable even the most timid person to gain confidence and build self-esteem. The horse instils self-awareness in those working with it, but also provides challenges.

The skills learnt whilst working with the horse are then transferred to other life skills, to enhance the progression of learning and increase independence.

The triangle

During riding sessions the therapist or instructor, the student and the horse form a triangle of learning. In non-riding sessions this triangle is repeated, but the horse may only be there in the person's mind. For example, during horse care and whilst mucking out, the horse may be out of the stable and in the field. The person is reminded to clean out the stable by doing a sequence of tasks involving taking out the dirty straw, sweeping the floor and putting clean fresh bedding in. They will then finish by laying the bed to prevent draughts, making it comfortable for the horse. To complete this, they need to empty the wheelbarrow and put the tools away safely, in the correct place. Throughout the performance of these tasks they will be reminded of how the horse needs its comfort and safety, as the person also does when resting. While they are going through the routine and process of this, the same thing will apply to them when making and setting fair their own bed, and tidying their room. The prompts will be made via the work they have done for the horse, so motivation for doing what was once a boring, difficult task now becomes more interesting and meaningful.

Here is an example of some everyday tasks that can be easily related to a horse:

Grooming	> Bathing/showering
Feeding	> Preparing own meals
Shopping for tack or rugs	> Shopping for clothing
Travelling to a show	> Travelling by public transport
Fitness routine for work required	> Fitness routine for work
Going to new places	> Leisure in the community
Training	> School or college

Other tasks may be related to the horses' relationships with each other, so sexual issues, friendships and family relationships, inappropriate behaviour in the herd, bad manners and bullying can be explored. In virtually every situation the use of EAT can be used effectively with positive outcomes.

In this way, there are always three equal elements in EAT: the therapist, the student and the horse.

The student learns how to interact with the horse, both in caring for the horse and in learning how to ride. The horse, specially selected and trained for this sort of work, responds to the young person's actions and commands. The therapist's role is to watch the interaction between the horse and the young person, and to help explain what happens in a helpful and authoritative way. By observing the student and the horse interacting with each other, the therapist can gain an understanding of the student, their needs and abilities, and can guide the student's learning by pointing out how the horse is behaving, and what that behaviour means. The student learns that, by changing their own behaviour, they can affect the behaviour of the horse.

For instance, on the first encounter between a student and a horse, the horse will usually want to sniff and nuzzle the young person. They should allow the horse to do this, and give it a gentle rub on the nose or pat its neck, while remembering to be calm and quiet around the animal, and to speak to it so it can recognise their voice. If they know the horse's name, then they should use it when speaking to it. A horse will take a lot of interest if the student has a carrot or piece of apple to offer.

A horse gets to know who feeds and talks to it. They like to be groomed so the next thing is to show the student how to groom it and which brushes to use and why. After a few meetings the animal will get to know the student's voice when they arrive and will prick up its ears and look pleased to see them. They will then start to learn the horse's unique body language from the way it responds to them. A horse's ears can tell the student a lot whether the animal is listening (ears forward) or defensive (ears back). If very relaxed the ears may be floppy. If the horse is anxious it may turn its back and put its ears flat back. Sometimes, one ear may be forward and the other slightly turned, to listen in all directions.

The horse loves to be praised so the student should always tell it when it has done well.

From the start, the young person needs to become part of the horse's daily routine: feeding, making sure it is well and alert, grooming, leading it out to the field, and mucking out the stable. Riding will form a part of the relationship, but it is not a necessary part. As long as the horse has food and water at the correct times of day, a clean bed, and plenty of exercise the horse will gradually form a good relationship with that young person.

When ridden, the horse will enjoy hacks with other horses and schooling exercises to help keep fit. The rider should take the role of leader of the horse and will need to learn how to be confident and calm with the horse at all times. The rider needs to learn what they can do easily to progress and then, when their muscles are able to do a little more, they can undertake more work. A horse should not be overworked, as being ridden and maintaining its balance over a long period of time will cause injuries and strains.

In this way, every aspect of EAT is a three-way partnership between student, horse and therapist, demanding awareness and responsiveness from each member of the triangle.

Holistic therapy: cognitive, psychological, physical

EAT encourages learning, enabling the student to learn through working with the horse and then to apply the skills learned to their daily lives.

The primary aim when working with those dealing with any kind of challenge, be it cognitive, psychological or physical, is to improve independent life skills. This is achieved by social interaction, working with the horse, and riding the horse, but a great deal of other learning inevitably takes place in the process of achieving this primary aim, in all sorts of ways and in a range of different situations.

Teamwork and the use of peers provide an excellent means of encouragement and good role modelling. The therapist may encourage a group of people to work together, to complete tasks with less support required than a one-to-one basis of learning. The rapport within the team should be fun and friendly, with everyone working together for one aim. By having at least one member of the team who can display good results, the others soon want to match them and become helpful team members. The therapist is able to support from a discrete distance and praise individuals for their roles as part of the functioning team.

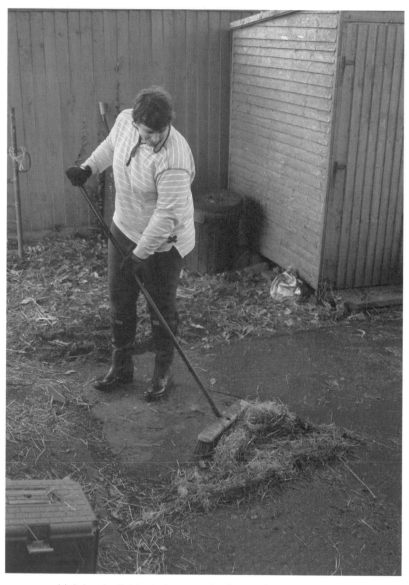

Helping individuals to grow in the work environment.

Improving personal skills happens gradually and cannot be rushed. Everything the student learns, from sweeping to putting a bridle together after a thorough clean, takes a little time. Many students have difficulty sweeping efficiently, but by learning to care for the horse and taking pride in its care, they learn how to ensure the animal's cleanliness. Once they have been able to learn the significance of being proud of their tasks they are able to transfer this pride to their own well-being. They then learn how to keep their own room tidy and are pleased with their work after cleaning tops and vacuuming.

A student will frequently be proud of completing their first journey on public transport, or managing their own budget and saving some money. One of the quickest ways to learn how to take pride is when they have helped to cook a simple meal, and the meal is appreciated by others.

Following on from this is taking responsibility, which means that they need to understand when something goes wrong and why it went wrong. It is a steep learning curve for someone to admit they have made a mistake so honesty is also part of the recipe for improving personal skills. With that comes problem-solving and decision-making. All of these can be learnt gradually through the work done with the horse.

Not everyone is creative, but with encouragement the student can learn to think creatively in ways that may resolve a variety of problems. When learning to feed they may realise that they could add the treat for their horse (an apple) into the feed, and ask if this is good for it.

Then when learning to bake a cake the student may think of similar ideas (chocolate) to go into their cake, or ideas for decoration. It is again up to the therapist to help the student think outside the box and come up with useful problem-solving ideas.

As already discussed, people don't come in discreet packages, with only cognitive challenges, or only physical challenges – each element affects the others, sometimes in unexpected and unforeseen ways, and this is why the holistic approach offered by EAT is so effective. But, of course, there can be questions of emphasis, where cognition is providing the main challenge for the student, or where psychological or physical difficulties are impeding their abilities in other areas.

EAT can be seen as providing enormous benefits in each area independently, as well as in all the areas taken together:

Cognitive therapy

Transferable skills can be used to a great advantage for personal development and life skills. These may be as basic as personal hygiene, or tying a shoelace. Feeding a horse may relate to eating a healthy diet, and a person may even learn to ride more assertively rather than passively. This assertiveness can then be transferred to social situations.

These primary aims can then progress to a more demanding skill level – like making more complex choices, leading to overall decision-making. Some clients can increase their skills to help prepare them for working and living in the community. Stable management and riding skills are increased, enabling them to improve their skills for the working environment.

Skills learned may include:

- to follow one-step instructions, like putting on a riding hat
- follow simple routines, such as getting ready to ride
- make choices between two items
- relate properly to others
- to keep safe
- take care of belongings
- take part in activities
- communicate through words and signs

Psychological therapy

EAT as an element in therapy in a psychiatric setting can bring extra value to a person's treatment in that it offers a better understanding of psychological functioning and motor skills.

It also raises questions of discipline and teaches assertive skills, which is ideal for those with problems in this area. General self-esteem is lifted and the therapist can reach a realistic view of the student's abilities.

The horse is valuable in enhancing the senses and emotions, and the horse's temperament can match or oppose the person's temperament. The horse may have a calming or a stimulating effect, which can increase self-esteem for people who have had inadequate relationships.

The psychological benefits are intertwined with the social and educational benefits, so through educational work, the person learns strategies to help them cope in difficult or frightening situations.

Having a secure and comfortable therapy area is vital for this treatment. Whether indoors or outdoors, the environment should offer privacy and be a calm, peaceful place.

Physical therapy

A person learns to improve and enhance their physical abilities by working with and riding horses. Other benefits include increased muscle, movement, tone and balance reactions. These factors assist and help to influence posture, which is one of the many aims of EAT.

The positioning on the horse is also important, as the transfer of the three-dimensional movement on the horse offers benefits such as decreased spastic muscle tone and increased hypo-muscle tone.

The holistic approach, embracing all three elements, increases benefits to those with physical difficulties to follow daily routines, and extend their range of skills.

For more severely disabled people, the stimulating effects of riding have proven to be of great value to the function of lungs, heart, circulation, and the digestive tract.

Goals for improving visual perception, space orientation, eye and hand coordination, rhythm and communication skills can all be integrated into the therapy.

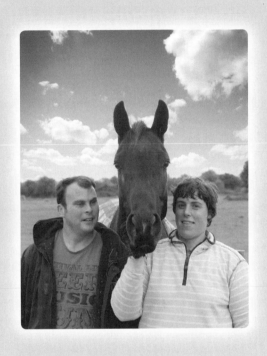

❧ Part two: ❧
Just a few of the challenges horses
can help with

Cognitive challenges

One of the most difficult things young people have to face is meeting new people and learning how to be friends. Friends talk to each other in sentences, laugh together and help each other; they listen to each other and go to places together, which they enjoy. If a person has a communication problem it becomes very difficult to socialise. Horses have a variety of ways of communicating, and this can help the student learn about the significance of body language. With encouragement, friendships are formed and good body language can be used to everyone's benefit.

Independence can be gained and lost throughout our lives. Some people can lose independence if hospitalised or kept in prison for a long time. They then become institutionalised and find it very difficult to manage outside of the institution. Many marriages form a dependence on their partner, and a spouse then finds it difficult if their partner leaves them or dies suddenly. We often tend to depend on our place of work and if we lose our jobs tend to drift and become depressed.

To gain independence a person needs to learn, or relearn, how to cope in society. With help and support, and by taking one step at a time and learning how to manage, a person can learn how to budget, cook or look after their own accommodation. They can practise shopping and travelling, coping with signs and symbols in the community. By using EAT, students can identify road signs when riding on the roads and learn how to work out amounts of food when preparing feeds for the horses. They gradually build confidence, by talking to others, and are helped to gain useful skills for helping them live within the community.

Often, despite having had a poor time at school, either in mainstream or specialist schools, young people start to excel when they feel they are achieving something. So, most goals have small steps to achieve, leading on to another, and then another. With encouragement and praise for gaining each small step, the student gains confidence and a heightened self-esteem. Most colleges and specialist schools now help the learner in this way. A small step is never too small, and can lead to greatness. Helping students to utilise their abilities rather than their disabilities, enhances their performance and progresses them to the next step more quickly.

We can liken this to the training of a young horse. A foal is weaned from its mother and turned away to 'playschool' with other young foals when it is old enough. Its mother will have taught it to graze for good grass and find fresh water, will have kept the youngster safe from harm from other horses, and will have shown it where to find shelter from the rain and the sun. The foal will have been with her when loud noises occurred, such as thunder or from vehicles, and learned the fight or flight reactions, although this is instinctive, the foal copies the reactions of its mother.

When at playschool with other young foals, the foal socialises and mixes with them, gaining new experiences, learning new lessons all the time, and some habits start to form: not always good ones for trainers.

Once the foal is about three or four years old, it is brought in to school. This means it will learn to be handled by humans and gradually get used to having weight on its back and a bit in its mouth. Once the foal has reached the stage of accepting a rider for a short time, it may be turned away for a winter to consolidate its schooling and have a rest, allowing its young bones to grow strong and healthy. This first schooling and handling by humans is similar to children's infant school. The young horse responds to the new environment, mixes with and sees other older horses behaving well when ridden, and is encouraged by an energetic tone of voice and praise when it has completed each small step well. Gradually, the foal learns to accept the saddle and bridle, and gentle slow movements by the rider. It learns to halt when asked gently and to walk on by using the rider's aids. By continuous repetition of these actions the foal comprehends and responds, and can then begin new experiences.

As a four year old, the horse is then brought back to school to continue its further education. Everything it learnt the winter before is re-taught and fine-tuned, so the horse has even better and quicker responses. Each day, it learns new things in movement, sound, sight and touch, with its senses vital for the animal's maturity and growth. The horse forms communication by using all of its senses and reacting to them. Any new movements – for example, jumping – are taught slowly and gradually, aiming to simulate what a horse would do naturally in the wild. Any youngster will naturally follow its mother and the rest of the herd to jump over a small log or hedge. The rider becomes the leader, so now the jumping has to be taught from a different viewpoint. Starting off with some loose schooling without a rider on its back, is one way of introducing this; following an older horse over a log when out on a hack is also helpful. Gradually, the young horse becomes used to the actions of the rider, and will work out its own way of jumping over poles or other jumps in its way.

Often, this is where many problems begin. Hormones can start taking over, or the horse begins to anticipate what the rider might ask. It may begin to change shape as it grows and the saddle may hurt at times. The horse may have an impatient rider, or other riders who are not so kind or consistent as its initial teacher, and it may resist or show signs of challenging behaviour. The horse will then need to go back to its initial training to re-establish good habits and aim for consistency in all its work.

This is not so very different from humans: correcting our negative views to positive, and changing our bad habits to good ones. Often, by changing the sequence of ways to complete a task, we can improve it. For instance, if a young person is used to eating their dinner in front of the TV, and leaving their plate on the side to be picked up, to start to change these bad habits, they need to change the sequence of events leading up to dinner. So, they need to start to help with preparing the table and the food, eating at the table with others, and clearing up after themselves. By doing this often enough, good habits are formed and replace the old.

Some people like to take control and can be very bossy or authoritative. The horse is a great leveller and will not accept forceful behaviour. I remember a girl who had Down's syndrome, who liked to tell everyone else what they should be doing and how they should do it. She tended to boast that she could do everything well, including riding. She was given a horse to ride who needed to be given the correct aids by a more experienced rider, but as she had professed to be a more experienced rider this should have been fine for her. However, when she tried to get the animal to do what she wanted, it refused and she became more and more forceful with her heels. She then became very frustrated and was advised to calm down and ask again, using a quiet gentle manner. The horse responded immediately to her better manners and she enjoyed riding such a well-mannered horse. This was definitely used again many times in other situations where she was guided to use good manners instead of being bossy, and her peers responded well to her asking nicely rather than shouting at them to do the task.

There were also times when she was very stubborn and refused to complete a task on the yard. Again, she was reminded of the way the horse had been stubborn, and how good it had felt when it had responded well to her. Whenever she was bossy or stubborn she was given that horse to ride, and each time, she felt more fulfilled and pleased with her progress when the horse responded to her gentle tone of voice and sympathetic aids. Her memory of how she interacted with that horse helped to change her attitude and lessen her stubbornness. She learnt how to become more sympathetic to others, and how to speak appropriately to gain a better reaction.

She was often asked to demonstrate how to do a task or a movement when riding, which gave her a sense of pride, tempered with a sense of realistic value when she found something too difficult. For example, she could ride a circle in walk, trot and canter, but when asked to do this without stirrups she would lose her balance and complete the circle in walk.

So the horse is able to teach us how to communicate better, not only with horses but also with other people. By helping the student to refine their aids to the horse, and by asking them to refine their tone of voice or manner when talking, they are more able to do this automatically. Often, some students tend to talk too quickly or are unable to pronounce some words correctly, and a way of helping them with this is through lunging the horse or loose-schooling.

Horses pick up on the tone and variation of a voice, so a timid person who cannot throw their voice learns to speak in a clearer more commanding manner. Someone who tends to speak in a monotone will learn to adjust their tone of voice to suit the horse's instructions. So, for instance, if a horse is trotting gaily around in a circle and one wants it to slow down to a walk, the command should be made in a lower tone of voice, with the sound of the word 'walk' elongated to 'WAAALLLKK'. Likewise, to increase pace, one would heighten the tone with a short, sharp 'trot on'.

Any other non-horse commands used would be meaningless, as the horse has been taught to respond to those words and tones. So for students who talk rather a lot, this helps them to be careful in choosing what to say, and to say it at the right time. People who talk a lot tend not to listen to others, and will miss some very obvious cues. The horse again helps here, as the person in the school with it will need to watch the horse's ears and its attitude for signs of anything that is likely to happen when it adjusts its pace. Quite frequently, the time for this is when the animal is asked to canter in a lighter tone, and it will buck in exuberance or may turn in to the handler instead of staying on its own path. The handler needs to use all their listening and observation skills to keep the horse in a steady rhythm of pace.

Away from the horse all communication lessons learnt with the horse are recalled to the student in other situations. So, for instance, if Bill is talking to someone else and Annie interrupts his conversation, speaking over him loudly, she can be reminded of the way the horse responded to her when she talked too loudly and was not clear. She now needs to consider Bill and listen to his conversation, just as she watches the ears on the horse to see if it is listening to her.

Peer groups play a large part in helping this along. When individuals have been through the same therapy with a horse, they will be more helpful, reminding their colleague to wait and listen instead of continually interrupting others.

When a person learns something, the quality of their life is improved because they have become a more effective individual. Why then, when an individual passes a course of instruction with high marks, possibly at the top of their class, do they remain an ineffective person? Is it possible that the individual in question never actually learned anything; they merely gathered information and remembered it?

Gathering information means exactly what it implies: gathering information. Learning is when a person consciously entertains an idea, becomes emotionally involved with that idea, and acts on the idea and improves their results. The bottom line is results.

Reading, remembering and repeating do not constitute learning. That concept may earn an individual a degree, but it will not necessarily make them an effective person ... at anything.

Let us take a salesperson as an example, although I could just as easily use a lawyer, a cabinetmaker or a secretary. A salesperson only closes one sale in twenty, so they are ineffective. However, a hypothetical salesperson attends a course on closing sales, and passes the course with flying colours. If asked a question on closing a sale, this person will answer it correctly. However, back in the marketplace they still only close one sale in twenty. They have learned nothing.

Learning is therapeutic and the process of learning can be extremely therapeutic, or it can be damaging. People with learning difficulties may take longer to learn something, they may copy bad habits and revert back quickly, but if learning is done consistently they will understand the prompting to remain on track until learning has taken place. A young horse can also lack confidence and find movements too difficult, so needs to take things slowly and have time to enjoy what is asked of it. An overconfident and naive horse may race along without due care, and if going too fast over its first cross-country course, could slip or fall and then be afraid of future cross-country courses. In the classroom we have seen young people like this: some so shy and quiet, never asking questions and afraid to put their thoughts to others; some who seem noisy, always guessing at the answers to questions and not caring if the answer is wrong. The ideal young person listens to the teacher and is able to answer questions when asked and will frequently get the correct answer. If they get the wrong answer, they are willing to find out where they went wrong in an effort to learn more.

Behavioural and psychological challenges

Kate suffered from depression and had attempted to take her own life on two occasions. Her parents had split up, but were concerned about her, and she was able to visit both whenever possible. She loved the horses and found that whenever she felt depressed she could go and hug a horse and talk the problem through with it. By keeping to the yard routines, she was able to hold back the noises in her head and focus entirely on the horse's needs. By focusing on her goals and working towards various qualifications, she managed to push depression away whenever it struck.

Kate was a good rider and enjoyed working towards dressage tests and simple showjumping. One of the ways to help her was to get her to concentrate on the next jump whenever she knocked one down. Instead of looking back at the knocked-down fence, she needed to look forward. This became a very useful analogy to be used at other times when depression took over, or when she perceived bad things had happened to her.

I love this analogy as when we have a knock-back in our lives, it is better to look ahead at the next step in our future rather than dwell on what is past and can't be changed. By perfecting our jumping technique and the training of the horse, we can aim for a clear round of jumps with fewer knock-downs. In the same way we can change or alter our own course for the future to find enjoyment in the things we do.

Many people who have been diagnosed with autism spectrum disorder or Asperger's syndrome focus on details, and are often extremely talented. They are the typical professor, who may have few words and seem to be in their own world, but can work out what is required to get someone to the moon. Usually, they are excellent with computers or technological items, good with numbers, or know every breed of horse and can identify them all. Helping these people to bring out their talents can increase their confidence and self-worth.

They need routine to work well, so working with the horse routine is ideal and meaningful for them. Each person has their own particular talent, and finding it is a useful way of guiding them for a future career. Such individuals are often very self-absorbed and do not show any empathy for other people's problems. However, because of their attention to detail, when working with the horses in the usual routine, they often report something that could be vital to the horse's welfare. They also find it very difficult to accept any changes to the routine, so need to have gradual changes made in order to form new routines. An example of this may be when a horse becomes ill and requires isolation, necessitating that the horse will be in a stable away from others; that all equipment for its welfare is kept separate; and gowns and boots are used by the staff when attending to it. For the person with Asperger's this means that the actual work tasks stay the same: the horse still needs to be fed and mucked out, but the way of doing this will change according to the infection.

Helping people with eating disorders is one of the most difficult problems to manage and understand. I can relate to someone who eats through a need for comfort or even obsession, but trying to comprehend the thoughts of a person with anorexia is nearly beyond the bounds of my perception. When a person weighing less than six stone, with their bones showing, says they are fat then what can we say to help them to be realistic?

Riding and working with horses tends to help a person to become more fit, agile and energetic. A person with anorexia is usually very agile and energetic as a result of living off adrenaline and stamina, and as we don't want them to lose more weight it can become a vicious circle. They also aim to work hard in order to lose their perceived fat body, but when they build muscle and become fitter they think it is fat and try to get rid of it. Another thing they tend to have is a heightened degree of interest in food and nutrition, and will happily go food shopping and look through recipe books for details of the food they intend to cook, and know more about calorie counting than anyone else. They can also usually guess other people's weight correctly and will have a good understanding of the horse's weight and appropriate food needs. It is their perception of themselves that is so distorted.

Jenny weighed in at below six stone and had been in hospital previously to help her become stable as her health had deteriorated drastically. She had a deep love of horses and wished to continue to ride and look after them. Initially she was very weak, needed a sheepskin pad to sit on over the saddle to prevent sores, and could only ride for a quarter of an hour, but gradually, she gained her strength over a period of time. We needed to encourage her to eat little and often, as we do with the horses when trying to get them fitter. She needed special care for her teeth so she was able to watch the horse dentist at work, to encourage her to look after her own properly. Her yard tasks involved less physical work but more challenging mental work, such as helping to prepare lessons for other students, recording and checking prices for new saddles and rugs, budgeting and making charts for the yard. She enjoyed taking photos and was given the opportunity to take some pictures of the horses in their beautiful summer coats, where she could see their conformation, and the splendour of their muscles rippling in the sunshine as they moved at different speeds in the fields. She also enjoyed music and liked to combine music with her riding. This combination of passions helped her to view things outside herself and focus on other beautiful things in her life.

Distraction techniques using the care of a horse can be helpful to people who self-harm, or who are recovering from addiction to drugs or alcohol. This can be done by monitoring their progress, and when signs of weakness occur, directing them to a task for the horse they love, which only they can perform at that time. It may not be helpful to suggest to a young girl who frequently cuts herself to use scissors for cutting the horse's tail, as she may take the scissors to cut herself secretly. However, that could also be the trigger for a change in her behaviour, as she would then be using a cutting instrument for a purposeful task that she may enjoy as much as cutting her own arms. To see her horse's well-cut, finished tail and be praised for it will help her self-esteem and contribute to further efforts to allay the desire to self-harm. This is a risk that may work out well.

Physical challenges

Lottie had been diagnosed with Prader–Willi syndrome. Children with Prader–Willi syndrome often have difficulties with coordination and balance from birth, owing to poor muscle tone. They have an insatiable appetite and unless carefully controlled will be extremely obese. They also may have moderate learning difficulties and challenging behaviour, especially where food is concerned. Usually, they are of short stature with small hands and feet. A fully independent life is not usually possible for people with Prader–Willi syndrome, but much can be done to help them to be as independent as possible in a sheltered environment.

Lottie had been known to eat from dustbins and would eat anything, including plastic items, if not prevented. She had a violent temper and would easily fly into a rage or try to hit people when food was an issue. If unsupervised, she would eat any food, including horse food, and as she never felt full could carry on eating to her death. However, she loved the horses and enjoyed riding. She gradually became fitter and more able to do tasks such as washing the horse down and putting on tack, which had been difficult for her. She enjoyed gymnastic exercises and was pleased to become quite proficient. She needed to adhere to the routine of the yard and was supervised at all times and at breaks, including lunch and dinner, where her intake was monitored carefully.

Lottie made friends and enjoyed her work with her peers. They helped her to be calmer when she felt angry, and would go with her to her favourite horse to talk and calm herself. Her parents were helped to find suitable specialist Prada–Willi supported housing for Lottie, which she now enjoys, while continuing regularly with her riding lessons.

Lottie had a rather extreme case of obesity, but many children and young people at present are overweight, and find it difficult to lose those extra pounds. A horse can bring a fundamental change to the routines and patterns in the life of an overweight person.

Anna weighed seventeen stone, was slow and lethargic and had moderate learning difficulties. She was unable to read or write or do any basic sums. She had been bullied at school and suffered from low self-esteem. She described herself as 'a useless lump' and felt she couldn't achieve anything, but she had a dream: she wanted to ride and work in a top event yard.

By helping her to set short-term goals and change her views of negative thinking to applying positive mental images of herself actually living her dream, she was able to make a start on a more achievable future. She then had to work hard to attain her goal of losing weight first, but she was smart and found ways to work that enabled her to lose weight, whilst improving her muscle tone and stamina. She kept to yard routines and had no time to pick at food or eat any snacks, and maintained a consistent regulated diet of eating smaller portions and fresh vegetables and fruit. Beginning with fast walks, she eventually started going for runs, and using a watch to time herself.

Gradually, she learnt to use her time for many tasks and was able to walk her horse for ten minutes, trot for ten, and then do short bursts of canter for half a minute at a time. She timed herself when mucking out, which initially took her two hours, until she managed to complete it in less than forty minutes from start to finish. She learnt to time her cooking and was able to check the food was cooked at the correct time. She also learnt how long the washing machine took to do a cotton wash and spin. As she lost weight, her other skills improved. She continuously set new goals and was able to accept when they did not go according to her plan. She did not accept defeat, but changed her plan to a new level of achievement. She was committed and persistent and started to believe in herself.

Many people with learning or physical difficulties struggle to dream. They may wish for something, but simply wishing is not enough to make things happen. Anna showed that by visualising herself with less weight and riding a good horse, she could start to dream the big dream. She reduced her weight to ten and a half stone, and gained the skills needed to aim for that top job.

One of Bill's difficulties was that he was unable to use his fingers well to write, draw or tie shoelaces. Through progressive work, putting a head collar or bridle on the horse, he began to use his fingers more effectively, and learned how to hold a pen and do up his shoelaces.

By looking at the achievements made by Bill in a fairly short space of time, we can see how his physical abilities improved, not only by doing heavy physical work, such as mucking out a stable, learning to use a fork, shovel and broom, and push a wheelbarrow, but also by helping him to use his fingers more effectively for fine motor coordination.

He gained further physical coordination when riding. It is not easy to mount or dismount at first, and most people find this cumbersome when they begin to ride. When the movements of the horse's paces are added it is a whole different ball game and can be very nerve-racking for the novice rider, let alone for someone who has difficulty with their own balance and posture. Each step is a major achieve-ment, and balance and rhythm become even more challenging when trotting. During this step, Bill was able to talk to the horse, stroke it and learn how to increase or decrease the speed by using his own body movements, which helped him to gain more confidence. He worked with a partner and in a team, and learned how to ask for help when necessary.

Bill not only gained improvements in his physical ability, but in-creased his communication skills, vocational ability and social skills. He learnt to identify basic feed charts and recognise amounts of different food to give, as well as how to use the scales to weigh hay. He also learnt how to adjust his behaviour in a variety of situations, such as controlling excitement or anger.

The educational, physical and psychological elements derived from the horse care and riding, related to Bill's own welfare. As a result, he was able to groom himself and dress appropriately; make his own bed; do his laundry and tidy his room; he was more able to shop and prepare his meals; he joined others in his leisure time and began to make friends; he gained confidence when answering the telephone and when asking for items to buy. He is now well on the way to becoming independent and needing less support.

Cathy was unable to push an empty wheelbarrow when I first met her. She was physically very weak and had spent most of her child-hood in hospital, having a variety of operations. She was also very timid and would not speak to anyone unless she was spoken to first. Her literacy and numeracy skills were poor, and she was very dependent on her mother. She loved the horses and wanted to be with them in her future. By working with them and learning to sweep the yard, muck out effectively and push heavy, full wheelbarrows, she gained in her physical achievements and her confidence grew. She did some regular gymnastic exercises (vaulting) on the horse, and rode quiet, safe horses initially. After three years, she was able to hold conversations with others, lead discussions, and explain to new, young people how to muck out or tack up the horse. She was able to look for and identify bus routes and, to find her way in familiar towns. She learnt how to cook simple meals and complete her own laundry, and was always very neat and tidy, so that was one area that needed no improvement. In addition, she learnt how to be safe around the horses and was able to point out any unsafe aspects, such as a rake left in the yard, in the way of people walking past. Cathy gained the confidence she needed but never became overconfident, and continued her progress in further education. She went to live in a supported house with other colleagues who enjoyed her company and had similar hobbies.

In some riding centres there is the opportunity for those with severe physical difficulties to feel the pleasure of the sun on their faces and the wind in their hair, by sitting in an open horse carriage, specially designed to take a wheelchair up a ramp so they can sit behind the horse. There are also specialist lifts that can lift a person onto a horse with ease. Whether riding or driving, the smile on the person's face makes it all worthwhile.

People with spinal malformation and curvature, or those who suffer from congenital muscular conditions may benefit from the close proximity of the horse, and the gentle movement of the horse's walking pace.

It is rare for anyone with epilepsy to actually have a seizure when they are riding a horse. Most people with epilepsy learn to manage well and accept that there are times when they will have a seizure. Learning to cope following a seizure, and helping other people around them to respond appropriately, is crucial. Quite often, the person will know what triggers a seizure and will be able to avoid it. I knew one young boy who was prone to them when he saw lines, such as lined paper, or railings in garden fences. Interestingly enough, some animals can sense seizures before they actually occur. Dogs are able to alert people of this and horses seem to know when something is wrong with their handler or rider. It is well-known that often more temperamental horses will be calm and passive when a disabled rider rides them, and will often sniff a person more than normal if something is not quite right.

There is a belief that a person who suffers from epilepsy is less likely to have a seizure during riding times, as they may be distracted from focusing on how they are feeling to what is actually happening with the horse beneath them. This may well prevent the problem from occurring. Distraction is a very helpful tool, especially for those with challenging behaviour or more severe difficulties. When the person is asked to consider something about the horse, it stops the chain of behaviour erupting into a full-blown explosion, and the person has time to calm down and to focus on more immediate tasks with the horse.

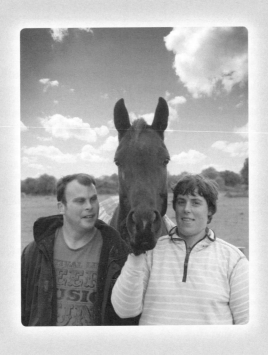

❧ Part three: ❦
Real people, real situations,
real changes

Being healthy and maintaining dignity

Self care and laundry

Every day, in the yard, there is tack to be cleaned after use. The care and protection of the leather is important to prevent sores on the horse, maintain the life of the saddle or bridle, and for good presentation. Saddlery is expensive, so thorough cleaning, oiling and leather protection are vital. Certain items can be washed by hand or in a washing machine, such as the numnahs (saddle cloths), boots and bandages, and light rugs. Bits and stainless steel parts are cleaned thoroughly, as are the stirrups.

When the student is doing these tasks, the care for the horse's harness and other equipment can be linked to doing their own laundry, with their daily underwear and clothing being put in a basket ready for washing. On an individual's laundry day they learn how to separate dark items from light and how to use the washing machine. Coats and jackets may need to go to the dry cleaner, like heavy horse rugs. Shoes and boots are encouraged to be cleaned daily, like tack cleaning, and made shiny for good presentation. Good presentation is necessary for going for job or college interviews, as well as for certain events such as weddings, funerals, and prize-giving presentations. So the analogy of the horse and rider collecting their prize after completing the competition or show is very useful, and a good habit to maintain, as they are expected to look smart and clean.

Another way of explaining good presentation is when eating out in a slightly more expensive restaurant, and seeing the way the table is laid, then aiming to do that in their own home. Many of those with special needs find it difficult to lay the table and put on a tablecloth. If a person is lucky enough to find a crease down the middle of the cloth it can then be likened to the riding school: 'The crease goes down the centre line, Bill'. This helped him to aim for equal sides on a rectangular table, as well as being useful when folding or ironing items. Bill has learned to understand and make use of the rectangular space of the riding arena when working with his horse from corner to corner across the centre point. By drawing the parallel between the arena and the tablecloth, Bill is able to understand how the tablecloth should be folded, and where the centre line should lie when folded out across the table.

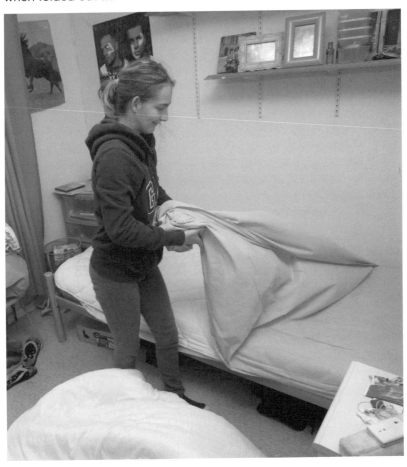

Learning life skills.

Joe was a young offender with an aggressive attitude and challenging behaviour. He used to steal, take drugs, and was frequently in fights. He had been taken into foster care at a young age, owing to a poor family background, whereby his mother had died when he was young and his father had left him to live with another woman. During his early teens he had mixed with a gang of youths that stole and bullied, and were often involved in fights with other gangs in the locality. Joe seemed to have no remorse or empathy with others' predicaments when I first met him.

For the first year, he was often angry and resistant to advice and suggestions, and did not want to mix with other young people. Initially, he appeared lazy when working on the yard and reluctant to do any tasks. However, he came to love handling and being with a particular chestnut mare. He started to learn the routine for feeding, grooming and mucking her out, and excelled in his work. It turned out that she was in foal, and Joe became even more attentive and careful with her. He was always calm around her and talked to her as she nuzzled him, looking for treats. He responded well to all the advice given by staff relating to this mare and her management, even to making suggestions himself. His attitude changed and he gradually became more mature and approachable. He learnt to ride on another horse with which he also showed a bond. In his riding he was very gentle and, at first, too passive, but he gradually learnt how to communicate with the horse through his own body movements, which he enjoyed, and derived satisfaction from the horse's response to him.

When the mare's foal was born he was thrilled to see the birth and followed the mare and foal's activities throughout his working day. He ensured the field was safe and free from all danger, that they had plenty of water and fresh grass to graze on and play in. In the evenings, he met his colleagues and was able to discuss the foal's activities and playfulness to them, laughing at some of the antics.

During this time, Joe became a responsible young adult and was able to communicate, without the need for aggression or poor behaviour. He took his role as groom for the mare and foal very seriously, and was able to care for and show his feelings to other people. Joe went on to achieve qualifications in Riding and Horse Care, and later found a job he enjoyed at a racing stud. He managed to save money and lived in a flat not far from his work, cooked and shopped for himself, completed his own laundry and paid his bills.

He had learnt to be independent and had no need to steal, take drugs or get into fights anymore. He even managed to find himself a lovely girlfriend.

Increasing choice and control

Coping with change

No one really likes lifestyle changes, but we have to learn to accept that changes are inevitable and part of life. Sometimes they are tinged with trauma or loss, or excitement and anxiety, and these often bring with them some behaviour changes for the person suffering the change. We tend to stick to our routines as a safety blanket, and whenever a student is going through a personal change in their life, I encourage routine work tasks to help them focus on the here and now.

The process of caring for another usually helps to focus on what is realistic, and to think positively about our own lives. Change brings opportunity and we need to see it to make choices about our future. If we miss the opportunity through worry or depression we may regret it later. Life should have no regrets. The need to continue on with usual routine when caring for the horse gives the chance to reflect on positive outcomes that may occur from the changes made in another part of their life. Small changes for some people become real challenges for others to overcome.

Angela found that small changes affected her and she became bad-tempered and moody. She found it difficult to accept constructive advice and answered people in a gruff tone of voice, muttering under her breath continuously. It could be a change to her usual laundry routine because the washing machine had broken, or a change to a planned outing because the bus was late. She would then talk about past illnesses of her relatives as though they had just occurred, as she remembered other sad changes to her life.

One way to help her with this was to allow her to understand the different changes a horse goes through during its day. If she spent time worrying about herself then the animal's feed would be late and the horse may be upset. If she was late for work, then the horse might not be ridden that day even though a lovely hack had been planned, so they would both lose out. If the horse wasn't groomed then it may get sores and would remain dirty. In addition, the horse's field mate was ill and needed to be stabled so the horse was alone for the day. The aim was to help her see that changes happen to both people and horses, and they need to be made the best of: for example, enjoying an unplanned outing more than the initial planned one; appreciating a new washing machine that works better than an old one; seeing the horse receive carrots in its late feed and watching it enjoy some time to itself to graze the best bits of grass without another horse pushing in. Gradually, Angela began to comprehend that not all changes were bad and from most, good things would emerge.

The funny thing about change is that we can accept it more easily if it derives from nature. For example, in the UK, the weather is always changing, so while we may decide to have a barbeque on Thursday, when it pelts down with rain we are happy to change the menu to shepherd's pie. We are grateful if we hear about earthquakes or other natural changes in other parts of the world, since we do not have to accept the difficulties that these bring. Politics is another area over which we have no real control: if the Government decides to make a big change to the education system, which won't start for three years, by the time it arrives, we have all accepted it, or they have moved on to another policy.

Most changes make us feel weak and unsure of where to go or what to do about them, as we lose a part of us that previously felt in control. If something happens to upset our usual routine, we flounder and become indecisive, struggling to regain the initial control that we perceived we had over our lives.

Now magnify that for a person who doesn't totally comprehend what is happening to their life when fear takes over. The horse can become their lifeline, their only stable point of reference. The horse contact can bring more strength and energy for that person in times of crisis or major change. The horse doesn't even need to do anything; it is just there, magnificent and strong, kind and affectionate; it doesn't change; is forgiving and loyal; the provider of unconditional love. The horse becomes the key to help the individual overcome the change and envision the positive aspects.

Making a positive contribution and improving quality of life

Hobbies and leisure

One of the difficulties many people have is not knowing what to do in their own leisure time, or not being able to do anything about providing for their leisure. Finding something we enjoy as a hobby is not always easy. However, when something is easy, we do tend to enjoy it more. When a person is doing a job they love and would enjoy as a hobby, as they learn more about it they often become more passionate, and more learning and pleasure occurs.

After hard exercise the horse is washed down and then turned out in the field with other horses to play and relax. The horse has learnt a lot during the exercise, and possibly fine-tuned its transitions from each pace, or practised its jumping skills. These are all skills the horse is able to do naturally, but by listening to the rider's aids and communication, and the very act of balancing itself with its rider helps with the horse's training. So a well-earned rest in the field with other animals is of paramount importance to recharge its batteries and consolidate the lessons learned.

This also applies to humans and, as we all know, too much stress is not healthy. Chatting with friends may be enough for some, or time alone to read or watch TV may be needed after a hard day mixing with others. Finding other activities can be stressful for a young person with special needs. Learning to socialise and mixing with the local community provides them with a wider range of choices and allows them to gain confidence with others. The thought that a horse needs to socialise and keep fit for its daily work provides an analogy for looking at sports or leisure centres, where swimming and gym facilities are available. Other sports may also be taken up via tennis or football clubs.

Hobbies and clubs may be found in the local library where books, films, and music may all be borrowed. Encouraging young people to use the facilities on offer in the community and helping them to gain access to them is vital for progression to independence.

John was overconfident and tended to think he could do everything well. He was often intimidating and patronising to others. Since he was quite good with his tasks in the yard and found it easy to answer questions immediately, with the correct answers, his work needed to be more challenging. As he completed his goals, he decided on new ones that he felt were achievable but different from any he had set before. For instance, he was able to travel independently to new towns by bus and train, but had never travelled by boat or plane.

One of his first goals then was to take a bus to the port and travel by boat to the Isle of Wight, which would then extend to a later project of travelling by plane to his home in Scotland. He became very excited at the longer-term goal and could see himself catching planes regularly to travel home. This led to a higher goal of managing his money and budgeting for these journeys. Of course, by looking at boat and plane routes and timetables, they became more meaningful and useful to him. He learnt how to use the Internet to check his banking and timetables, so became quite proficient in the use of a computer.

When riding, he was able to master the basic school movements on the school horses, but wanted the challenge of competing in a dressage test on a particular temperamental, thoroughbred mare, who was known to be quite strong, wilful and more difficult to ride. Working with her was quite a challenge, which mirrored his intimidating communication with others. He was unable to intimidate her and found that by making the ride fun and interesting, she began listening to him and responded in a better way. He completed the dressage test competition after a few months of practice, by forming a good bond with the mare. John is now able to stop himself from intimidating others, and can share a joke or an interesting conversation with them instead.

Many of the horses are taken out to local competitions, and when they go, safety precautions for driving horses need to be taken into consideration. The first thing is that they all should have a passport. This is owing to the restrictions made to prevent the sale of horses for consumption. However, we can liken this to young people obtaining their own passports, and give guidance on filling in the forms. The young people also need to be aware of the lorry or trailer's insurance details, MOT, and the amount of petrol or diesel needed. A calculation can also be made for how much money is required for the outing, including paying for entries and food needed.

This can then be compared and related to the person going on holiday, or for a day out. This sounds a little complicated, but the work is all in the preparation for the outing, which should hopefully be enjoyable.

If we consider what is required for an outing with a young child or baby, that is similar to what is needed to prepare for a horse. Not only are the vehicles checked for safety and up-to-date documentation, but the horse needs safety boots, rugs, saddle, bridle, and other items of saddlery, such as different bits for the bridle or a martingale. The rider needs the correct clothing, which includes hat, boots, jodhpurs, jacket, shirt, tie or stock, gloves and whip. Then, there is a first aid box, food for the day for the people, and food for the horse, plus water containers, not forgetting extra money and competition documents. Other factors to be considered are the weather and the need for extra clothing, for both horses and humans, if wet and cold.

We try to keep this simple. If Jane is going on holiday with her friend for a week, she will need help to complete the passport form and get it signed on time to have the passport for her holiday. She is then learning about time in terms of weeks, months and days. She needs to ensure she has the correct clothing for the holiday, so may need to go shopping for some items. Alongside this is her budget for the holiday, ensuring she can pay for her flight and accommodation, including any insurance. As it gets nearer to the time, she will probably need to book in online for her flight and to keep all her documents to hand, in a safe place. Jane will pack her clothing and toiletries neatly, and in order of probable use. Then she will have to weigh her bags, in order to check she is within the required weight limit. She may want some magazines for the flight, and should keep her flight, hotel and passport documents and purse in her hand luggage. Now she is learning about the time in minutes and hours.

How many different areas are there here for learning related to travelling with a horse? Of course, the experiences Jane will have at the airport are going to be new and challenging; meeting and talking to people; reading the flight times from the board; checking in luggage and having it weighed; and the actual flight itself. In fact, reading the departure board is very similar to reading the scores a horse gets when competing. Jockeys need to be weighed and checked before and after their ride, so again, there are more comparisons that can be used to make the situation more meaningful.

Families and relationships

There are few of us who haven't had the occasional problematic relationship in our lives, and, where there are other challenges in play as well, those relationship difficulties can sometimes seem impossible to understand or resolve. Observing how horses interact, and learning how to interact with them effectively, provides valuable lessons for the student in how to manage their own relationships.

Usually, in a group of horses, there is one horse who is the leader, who will always make sure they get their food first – and who will eat the others' food as well if they can get away with it! Their behaviour has to be managed in order to ensure that every member of the group gets what they need. In a similar way, students can learn to manage their own behaviour, to be aware of the needs of others, and to be open and responsive rather than self-centred and aggressive.

When Joe first heard about the death of his beloved grandfather who was the only person in his family to visit him, he was distraught and didn't know what to do with his life, as it seemed to have come to an abrupt end. By steering him to look after the mare and her foal and keeping to his work routine, he managed to get through the sad days. He spent time with the mare, watching the beauty of her behaviour with her foal: how she protected the youngster and nuzzled it away from danger; how she nourished with her milk and showed the foal how to graze the best grass. Joe was grateful when the mare allowed him to stroke the foal, and felt honoured to be able to do this. He later decided that he wanted to work with horses at a stud farm, and aimed to attain the necessary qualifications. The mare helped him to see past his sadness and start to make positive choices for his future.

Jake suffered from ADHD: he was very quick in his actions but not very efficient with tasks, as he usually needed to go back to finish off a task adequately. He was keen to have a girlfriend and met someone who responded well to him. However, the need to ensure that he knew about contraception was extremely important, as he would have found it difficult to manage his life with a partner and baby at such a young age, and it was apparent that he would have followed his sexual instinct without any thought for the consequences.

When a mare is taken to stud to meet a stallion she is swabbed and checked first for any infection. This example is helpful to describe the use of condoms and the prevention of sexually transmitted diseases.

The behaviour of a mare in season can be related to menstruation and the behaviour often associated with it when it occurs. This can be linked to hygiene and personal care when having a period.

However, the behaviour of the stallion when trying to mate with the mare is also a very useful point to pursue and discuss with both females and males. Usually, there is a sense of shock when watching a stallion mount a mare. This shock can be used to great effect when advising and cautioning about unwanted or inappropriate sexual behaviour, or bullying.

One of the most disturbing ways that love is shown from a human to a horse is after the young person has been previously abused by someone they love. Mary was abused as a child by her father, whom she loved. Since the horse needed her for everything to make it comfortable, she was able to love it as she had her father: she yearned to be needed. This can cause other problems, as often the person who has been abused becomes fascinated with putting their fingers in the mouth, nose and anus of the horse, which may lead to an unexpected response by the horse. Supervision is required at all times in such circumstances, and a healthy attitude to feelings of love needs to be established. Learning to respect other people's space is advantageous in making friends and forming relationships.

As our riding centre is situated so close to the New Forest, we see many new foals arrive in springtime, and this is thus an ideal opportunity to discuss the sexual behaviour of horses and of humans. Usually, the stallion can be recognised near the herd, and mares in foal are easily identified. The protection provided by other mares near the youngsters can also be seen, so family relationships can be explored and issues discussed, arising from problems that have occurred in a young person's childhood. Many people with certain special needs have the same sexual instincts and feelings as other people their age, even though their limitations may cause them to be similar to a much lower age group in many respects. Bill, for example, has been estimated to have a mental age of a six-year-old child, but has the natural urges and feelings of a man. This makes people with special needs extremely vulnerable to abuse and some inappropriate behaviour problems.

Interestingly enough, there are current discussions about whether to teach five-year-old children about sex education. This seems to be a good case for fieldwork and seeing nature at work. Young children who are sons or daughters of farmworkers see this first-hand, from a very young age. The mating of cows or pigs, and then the arrival of offspring, are natural occurrences for them: sex education at a primal level!

Staying safe

Taking risks

Many people with physical or learning difficulties are protected by their parents and carers from taking too many, if any, risks, but as they get older they need the challenges that risk-taking brings. Instead of thinking so much about their lower mental age, we must prepare them for adulthood and further independence despite that. Working with horses is very risky and injuries do occur, but as students they are supervised in the workplace and learn the safest ways to handle the horses and equipment. Riding itself is a huge risk for anyone, so risk assessments are completed thoroughly.

There are risks throughout our lives, but if we don't take them we will never be challenged to do anything. For young people with special needs it is important for them to have as many life experiences as possible, to ensure a good quality of life. A doctor will recommend any specialist therapy and inform of any major problems that could occur. Some may require the help of a physiotherapist or speech therapist, or another type of therapy needed. The risks are not just with the horses though, and if we look around our homes and in the community we can find many risks of which we need to be aware and prepare for, but by providing the opportunity to learn basic health and safety aspects, and by using the safety procedures consistently, risks can be reduced.

Some of the ways to reduce risks when riding are simple things, such as: always putting stirrups up until you actually mount the horse; making sure you walk round the front end to prevent being kicked; not offering titbits in your hand, to prevent bad habits of biting or pushing; when in the yard, keeping equipment in the correct place; hanging hay nets with quick release knots; putting water buckets down with the handle away from the horse, to prevent it being caught in it; leading and handling with gloves on; turning the horse away from you rather than towards you; and being aware of spooky items that may cause the horse to spook, for example, black bags or something not in the usual place.

In the home, simple procedures form good habits for safety; for instance: always checking that gas is turned off after cooking; keeping dangerous chemicals out of harm's way; and locking doors when going out and last thing at night. Other good habits are: ensuring that crockery, utensils and kitchen equipment are cleaned thoroughly to prevent food poisoning or infection; checking expiry dates on items of food; and ensuring that the fridge is the correct temperature. All of these daily, routine, good-practice habits also aid learning in other areas. Being able to identify expiry dates, checking temperatures and reading labels are all positive aspects of literacy and numeracy.

There is never a 'no-risk' situation when working with people and animals.

Safety in the community

The simple act of crossing a busy road can be really challenging for some. Safety in the community and learning to keep themselves safe are essential for vulnerable people. An awareness of fraud and exploitation is of increasing importance in today's world, so guidance when withdrawing money from a cashpoint, and when walking with bags or full purses is provided by giving advice, suggestions and prompting. Riding or leading a horse on the roads can be dangerous, and many sessions provide riding and road-safety practice, which can lead to a qualification. This helps to teach good road sense and enables the young person to recognise signs and markings when out in the community.

Part of Bill's work role meant he needed to do field maintenance and check the fields for safety when turning the horses out. He cleared the droppings as part of his daily routine and checked the water supply was plentiful. He also checked the fences to ensure they were taut and intact, along with the gate and any posts, and inspected the fields for litter or pieces of glass, to prevent the horses from sustaining any injuries. In addition, he looked for any poisonous plants, and was able to identify several and pull them out. He learnt the correct way to turn a horse out to grass, and be aware of other horses in the field. He also discovered the difficulties of feeding hay or feeds to several horses in the same field, and formed a routine way of managing them safely, and of keeping himself safe.

Bill then practised the same things when out in the community: looking for dangers and ways to keep safe when crossing the road, when going to shops or looking to buy items he liked or needed. He began to observe safety road signs he had learned and recognised when riding. Other safety observations he made were when he was eating in the café, with regard to fire exits, food poisoning and cleanliness procedures.

In the context of EAT, awareness starts with learning about horses. Anyone who is near a horse becomes aware of how big or friendly it is, and one of the first things that needs to be learnt is how big its feet are! Horses are very likely to tread on toes, so we help students become aware of this and teach them how dangerous it could be to stand behind a horse.

Learning how to be aware of dangerous situations takes time, and sometimes occurs through trial and error. Occasionally, the students learn best if they make a mistake in a supported environment, before going out in the big wide world. Health and safety awareness is a main part of their learning, and this becomes daily practice.

Vulnerability and exploitation

Horses can be very vulnerable and rely on humans for their safety and welfare: they can be ill, suffer from disease or inherited problems; they may be injured or suffer from panic, anxiety or stress-related illnesses.

One of the most important factors of horse care is the prevention of illness and injury. Safety factors on the yard and when riding are emphasised continually. Horses can shy at the smallest paper bag and can injure a leg meaning it will be unable to work for a period of time, and may need a vet, which is very costly. I will never forget a lesson I learned once when I dismounted from my mare and she caught her reins in her front leg, which panicked her. As the rein tightened it meant she could only go round in circles, panicking her even more. Luckily, she came to no harm, but the shock was enough for me to reinforce always using good habits by keeping reins held high enough not to loop around the horse's foot.

It is imperative that good habits and the formation of them is maintained and used consistently, to prevent a lackadaisical attitude and injury to the horse or person. There are always going to be times when accidents may occur – we cannot keep our horses or ourselves, wrapped up in cotton wool – but if we strive to be aware of any possible potential accidents then we can reduce them to a certain extent, and raise greater awareness of potentially dangerous situations.

By giving our young people the opportunity to protect the horses as much as possible, while also enabling the horses to have a good quality of life, in order for them to reach their potential, we are able to link this to the young people's own lives: they are able to learn how to care for the horse to prevent injury or illness, as well as learning how to do the same for themselves. A horse with a leg wound that needs cleaning and dressing daily is a responsible task, to prevent infection and help the healing process. Such responsibilities are encouraged and risks may be taken to promote that feeling of responsibility. The instructor must be able to trust that person and quite often will need to show this trust and help the young person gain self-responsibility.

Many horses are able to sort themselves out when jumping a course of jumps. If they knock one down, through either taking off too early or too late they learn to cope and work out their own striding for the next jump with little help from the rider. Most times, it is the rider's interference that causes the mistakes. The rider guides the energy, speed and the turns, but should give the horse freedom over the jump, then praise lavishly when the horse makes the effort. Next time, the horse may go clear as it has gained valuable experience.

Achieving economic well-being

Money management

Bill would quite often go on a walkabout by himself when he went shopping. He was given the responsibility of going to certain shops with a friend, and arranged to meet up with me at a set time. The trouble was he left his friend and went to the nearest phone shop to buy the latest mobile phone. He had a contract for an iPhone at the time, but wanted to upgrade to the new iPhone. As he had also been entrusted with his cash card, he had the necessary means to pay for it. However, he did not understand the contract charges or how much money the new phone was going to cost him. In his view, he just paid with a card and then had a new phone, the same as his friend.

To help him understand the concept of money he needed to not have too much available money to spend on luxury items. He didn't know the difference between £10 and £1,000, and had spent a huge amount of money previously on items he didn't need, which we then had to try to have refunded, as he just collected items he already had. Giving him a stricter budget and trying to sell his old iPhone was proposed. He also handed his card over for safe-keeping in case he was tempted again, which he was happy to do. There is a fine line between being responsible and being vulnerable, but the aim to strive for higher responsibility should always be there.

The boy mentioned earlier who suffered from epilepsy started using unlined paper to prevent the lines triggering a seizure, but he was given the responsibility of going out to the local town with his colleagues, with support at the end of the phone. He planned ahead and worked out the route and where they would go for lunch. However, he had a seizure and it transpired that he had been walking down a road with iron railings on either side. Prior to this, he had enjoyed his outing. He later felt a much greater sense of independence and self-responsibility, as he became more able to go out with friends, and found ways to solve his problem.

Looking at ways to get round problems and planning ahead enable greater self-responsibility, and lead to a less dependent lifestyle.

Coping when something goes wrong is a beneficial learning tool.

Bill caught a train to his home and was used to the routine of having to change trains at Southampton. He knew the platform he needed to go to for the next train. However, one day, there was a delay and the train journey had to be continued by bus via a different route to Southampton. He was able to keep in touch with me on his phone and explain what the problem was and how he was coping with it. He managed to arrive at Southampton by bus, and find the correct platform in time for his next train.

Work experience and finding a job

While performing everyday tasks for the horse, the student with special needs gains specialist knowledge of horse management, which helps them to gain useful future skills for work or voluntary work, and helps them to remain interested in the type of work they choose. The student may decide that the work in winter is too hard and choose to do a more sedentary job, but they will have learnt that they need to keep occupied, and how to look after themselves with less and less support.

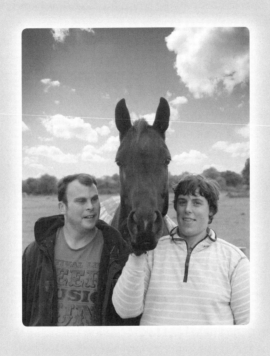

❧ Part four: ❧
The mind can do so much

Shaping behaviour

Whenever horses are ridden or handled, we are training them. Whether it is standing still in the yard, or performing a dressage test to music, we need a clear way of communication to be effective, and so need to understand how behaviour-shaping works. Firstly, we need to provide a stimulus; when the horse responds to our stimulus, we reinforce the response by either positive or negative reinforcement. Positive reinforcement encourages repetition of the response if it was the desired response, and negative reinforcement discourages the response if undesirable. Through this process, a non-verbal language is developed.

If we give the stimulus for walk to a young horse by using our leg movements, and it walks forward then we should praise the horse and relax the leg aids. However, if it doesn't walk, then we repeat the leg aids more vigorously. The relaxation of pressure from our legs and verbal praise becomes the reward, and the horse will want to do this again. The negative reinforcement is the more vigorous pressure, until it walks forward and gains praise.

A child who is asked to eat up their dinner may be praised for eating it, but if they throw a tantrum and throw the plate across the table they may receive negative reinforcement by sitting on the 'naughty step' until they have calmed down, which should discourage the behaviour from happening again. Of course, this does not always happen immediately and may take a period of time for the effects of positive or negative reinforcement to be noticeable. Any inconsistency in the giving of positive or negative reinforcement will slow up the process, so it must always be the same.

Gradually, the young horse is able to respond positively to more signs from the rider, developing a larger vocabulary with less use of any negative reinforcement.

Many people and animals have had poor behaviour responded to with positive reinforcement, which then creates more poor behaviour. How do we change this around?

I can think of a classic situation with a child who refused to eat certain foods. They were then rewarded by being offered food that they would eat; ice cream, for instance. The child quickly picked up that if they refused their dinner they would be given ice cream. You can imagine what happened at every dinner time after that. Quite often, instances like this are caused innocently by a caring parent who just wants the child to eat something.

Another instance could be a child who becomes ill and needs a lot of comforting and love from their parents and a day off school. This is normal, but what happens when the child discovers that every time they say they have a tummy ache they do not have to go to school and get extra attention from their parent? Boundaries need to be set and the help of a person outside the family, such as a doctor checking the child and pronouncing them fit for school, may be the way forward in this instance.

Horses too are very quick to catch on to our innocent failings. Children who ride are reminded to praise their ponies to aid positive reinforcement, but trouble may occur when they praise them all the time, even if the pony has not done anything worthy of their praise. So, when they are trying to catch it, the naughty pony trots away, even though they are still saying, 'Good boy, come here', so the pony thinks this is a great game, as it is being praised for trotting away. Frequently, the best thing is to ignore the bad behaviour, walk away and when the pony or horse is consumed with curiosity, or anxious not to miss a feed, it will come to be caught and will then be praised.

Rewards for positive reinforcement for the horse can be verbal praise, a pat or scratch on the neck, a rest or finish of the schooling session, or in the form of a treat, such as an apple or carrot. Negative reinforcement may be the absence of the reward, the repetition of the exercise, or stronger, clearer use of communication aids. Similarly, this can be applied to people.

Horses are our teachers, therapists and psychologists. They help us to respect their boundaries, and can provide positive reinforcement or negative reinforcement to the rider or handler. They can help us become consistent with our language and use of body movements, by responding at the right time and in the correct way, providing us with positive reinforcement. The horse will not respond appropriately if the rider is frustrated, too passive or lacking in concentration, and so becomes the psychologist, only responding in the desired state when the rider has calmed down or asks in a satisfactory manner.

When faced with changing behaviour and enhanced learning I think of this easy ABC:

- **A** is the *antecedent*: what happens leading up to the behaviour.
- **B** is for the *behaviour* itself, which may be the desired behaviour or undesirable behaviour.
- **C** is for the *consequence* of the behaviour.

An example of this could be Bill becoming more and more excited owing to his impending journey home (the antecedent), clapping very loudly and shouting (the behaviour), and spooking a horse tied up in the yard, which then breaks free from the tie ring and knocks its handler over (the consequence).

However, if we intercept the antecedent by distraction and ask Bill to fetch his grooming kit to help groom the horse, and remind him to be quiet on the yard (A), he will then go quietly and calmly to fetch his grooming kit (B), and the horse will remain calm while being groomed (C).

Of course, we cannot guarantee that we will catch the antecedent in time to change the behaviour and consequence, or we may not know what is triggering the behaviour, but if possible, being aware of and intercepting A or B will change C.

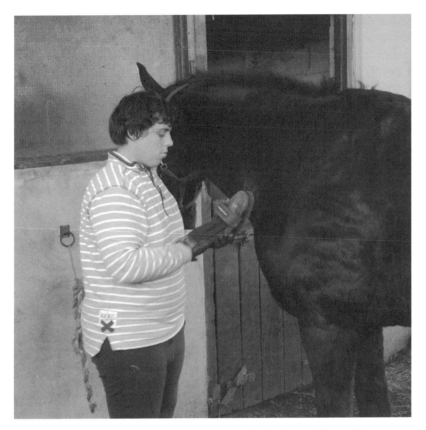

Grooming a horse can be used as a behavioural distraction.

The power of the mind

Developing a positive mental attitude is not easy for anyone, but we can strive for it. I imagine a paintbrush inside my head wiping away any negative thoughts I have, then replacing them with a positive thought, however small and insignificant it may seem. For instance, if I think that I will fall off at a particular jump I probably will, so I quickly replace that with the thought of clearing it with good balance, and seeing myself looking at a special marker, such as a tree in the distance, to keep my horse's line straight. I have then found a smooth way over the jump, trained the horse to keep a straight line and focused on my balance and the distant tree, instead of on falling off.

Many people who lack confidence need to be encouraged to change their way of thinking, and need to be with people who will encourage them to look ahead, and find the good in every difficult situation.

A lovely lady I knew was diagnosed with multiple sclerosis. Previous to this she had been a high-flying lawyer and was used to working in sharp suits and killer heels, and had never considered riding horses. When I met her, she had begun to ride with Riding for the Disabled, but was paralysed from the waist down. She wanted to continue riding and work towards competing in dressage tests. I was fascinated that although she had no use of her legs she was very relaxed, and the natural movement of the horse enabled her legs to touch in all the right places to give slight aids. This meant that she was able inadvertently to give the horse the signals to go forward naturally. Her upper body movements were practised to enable her to be completely relaxed and show little tension, while her upper back was supple, allowing her to use her back to provide correct signals to the horse. She bought her own horse, which was very well-trained and started competing, and a few years later won with her horse at the Paralympics. It was such a huge achievement for her to find a new lifestyle and love it enough to aim for the Paralympics and win!

I met a young man in his early thirties who was keen to ride in polo competitions. When I first saw him he was leaping on to a horse from the ground and could ride well at speed, in an easily controlled manner. I later found out that he had lost a leg mid-thigh, as a result of suffering from polio as a child. With an artificial leg, which wasn't noticeable, he strived to learn polo and played internationally.

Visualisation and relaxation

Both of the people mentioned above were able to visualise themselves actually doing what they wanted to achieve. Firstly, they found something they enjoyed doing, and established a love and passion for their horses. They set goals with achievable steps up the ladder to the highest goal they desired. They didn't rush up the ladder, but took their time with each step, perfecting it with minute details of learning and physical improvement, all the while keeping that highest goal in their mind. They pictured the end goal, seeing themselves on the podiums collecting their prizes, patting the horses and hearing the spectators cheer, and used all their available senses to bring the images into focus and feel the emotion of winning. They learnt relaxation techniques to help relax and contract muscles, and to help breathing, which also helped the images be clear for the subconscious mind to act on.

They used clear positive words when riding, and if difficulties arose would find the right words to use, to change a negative situation into a positive one. For instance, if the horse spooked at a flowerpot near the marker in the dressage arena, instead of dwelling on the spook and saying to themselves, 'now we've messed up the whole test, and we won't get such good marks', the comment to themselves would be, 'what a quick recovery from that spook, now we are really showing an amazing canter'.

They also followed the 'as if' principle, as in psycho-cybernetics, riding in competitions as though they had already gained their end goal. This showed increased confidence and heightened their self-image so that they looked and felt as if they had already succeeded.

My students may not have these aspirations, but having discovered the 'hook of the horse', they too are passionate and grow more motivated to succeed in whatever sphere they choose. They are on a stepladder to their own success, whether that is managing to ride a horse in walk, living in a house with two friends, or completing the British Horse Society exams, and finding a job they like.

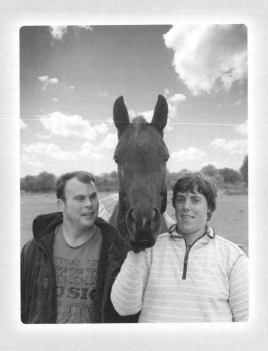

❧ Conclusion ❧

Conclusion

So what has happened to Bill and his colleagues?

Bill is still working on a voluntary basis with horses, and at a local farm with other animals. He is progressing well by becoming more independent, requiring only supportive prompts and some help with literacy and numeracy. He has a social life and meets friends at a club and in the pub. His motivation for progress remains strong through his relationship with the horses. Some of his colleagues have gone on to further education colleges and some like Joe have progressed to acquiring paid employment and living in supported lodgings or in rented accommodation. They continually update their goal plans and work consistently towards their new goals.

You can clearly see that Equine Assisted Therapy offers many benefits that lead to a more rewarding life. It is effective and provides another hope or chance for people with disabilities and their families. It mixes sport, fun and the gymnastic ability with education. It heightens the senses, increases physical abilities and produces higher levels of communication. It creates confidence and powerful feelings of self-worth. Importantly, it can help them find a desirable and good quality of life and hope for their future.

For many children with disabilities or learning difficulties the things they take note of, or are more interested in, will be apparent at school or at home. Quite often, they will shine when they are drawing or painting, or they may like games such as football or board games. When the parent or teacher realises that a child likes doing something, they often use that to promote further interest. If a child likes pictures of horses then that could be channelled to further learning and therapy. In helping children gain as much experience as possible, parents may take the child to learn to ride, or be with ponies at local stables, or may join Riding for the Disabled Association (RDA) for fortnightly sessions, for a period of time in the UK. This is often a great start for them, and so the love of the horse begins.

For continued therapy and progress, and with a view to the young person or school leaver gaining more skills, in order to learn to become more independent, they are often referred by teachers, the RDA, social workers or other services to specialist residential colleges or supported day care. Unfortunately, in the UK at present, there are few residential colleges that use Equine Assisted Therapy. However, with more supported housing and private residential care facilities incorporating farms or smallholdings, stables, or small animals, there is the opportunity for a person with special needs to be directed to an appropriate placement of their choice.

Equine Assisted Therapy will open new doors for both the person with difficulties and for their families and friends.

How to access EAT

Colleges of further education

Colleges of further education now also provide qualifications that are similar to, or complement the British Horse Society (BHS) examinations. Many of the students with difficulties strive towards gaining some of the Level 1 and 2 qualifications. For some, it is a way of helping them gain more confidence as they progress through the steps; for others, it may be a way to help them on a career path for the future. Some will be pleased to have achieved one or two steps of the list of tasks to be learnt. The horse gives them all a meaningful and pleasurable way of learning, which is therapeutic in itself.

Many equine or agricultural colleges offer a variety of equine courses at differing levels of ability. National Vocational Qualifications (NVQ) are also used to help people take steps up the qualification ladder. Many agricultural colleges also provide NVQ and BHS courses.

It is a good idea to check with your local college and find out which courses they have available, where there is some one-to-one support for the learner.

Specialist colleges

The Fortune Centre of Riding Therapy

This is ideally for sixteen year olds or over, who have completed their schooling and are looking to gain further independence whilst working alongside the horses. It is a specialist college and consists of a three-year residential course of therapy and education for young people with disabilities.

www.fortunecentre.org

Residential care

Other support may include small farms or smallholdings, which may work closely with animals as therapy for people with special needs. This may be on a daily basis, or provide residential care for those people who need far greater support on a daily basis. The residence is required to be registered with the Care Quality Commission, and available options need to be discussed with a social worker. There are also some specialist types of residential care for specific syndromes or disabilities: eg. autistic spectrum disorders, Prada–Willi syndrome.

Supported lodgings/shared lives

Supported Lodgings with Equine Assisted Therapy can be found widely in the UK. The best source of information is to contact your local social services, to find out if there are any in your area, or speak to your young person's social worker. The centres will be expected to follow an individual care plan, according to the person's needs, which can be related to the learning they do while working with horses or other animals.

Many places offer support with the horses by qualified staff on-site and provide other opportunities for voluntary work or work experience of the student's choice, while they are receiving benefits. Some may progress to paid work or may wish to continue their education at a college or as part of an apprenticeship.

Helpful organisations

British Equestrian Vaulting

I have mentioned vaulting as being gymnastic exercises on the horse which helps with many skills especially physical development. They have groups in Scotland, England, Wales and overseas.

www.vaulting.org.uk

Riding for the Disabled Association (RDA)

This may be your first port of call to find out if being with horses could be helpful for your child, or a disabled person. There are groups around the UK and volunteers, who are extremely knowledgeable.

www.rda.org.uk

The British Horse Society (BHS)

This is the place to find books and articles that may be helpful for the young person learning about the care of horses. They also provide qualifications towards good practice of horse care and riding.

www.bhs.org.uk

The Pony Club

You don't need to own your own pony to join, and children can meet new friends and learn while they are having fun. They provide tests leading up to BHS examinations and this is also a great place for books and pony related items.

www.pcuk.org

LEAP

Equine Assisted Facilitated Psychotherapy and training.

www.leapequine.com

Federation of Horses in Education and Therapy International (HETI)

Global organisation that connects people with other countries, centres and individuals who offer equine-facilitated activities. It also helps develop new programmes worldwide.

www.frdi.net

Holistic Equine Assisted Relationship Transformation (HEART) Centre, Surrey

A form of equine assisted therapy with holistic coaching. Has programmes to support individuals through relationship or confidence issues and has facilities to support more challenging conditions as well.

www.equine-assisted-therapy.com

Strength in Horses

A team of clinical psychologists together with equine specialists using their understanding of mental health and horses to help promote wellbeing.

sihequinetherapy.org

Horses Help Heroes

Individuals using their knowledge of horsemanship to support, both physically and mentally, British servicemen and women who need help to live active and fulfilled lives.

www.horseshelpheroes.org.uk

Help for Heroes

Books and information for people who have had traumatic injuries.

www.helpforheroes.org.uk

Eagala UK

Founded in 1999, the Equine Assisted Growth and Learning Association (EAGALA) is the leading international non-profit association for professionals using equine therapy (horse therapy) to address mental health and human development needs.

www.eagala.org/UK

Fetlocks Housing, Dorset

Supported housing community where young people may learn life skills such as: finance, health and fitness, social behaviour, educational skills for training and employment, and many other relationship-building skills.

www.fetlocks-dorset.co.uk

Bodster Equine Assisted Learning Centre, Ryde, Isle of Wight

Jo and Giles Boddington offer equine assisted learning by working with anyone young and old, including those with complex needs such as Autism, Aspergers and Downs.

www.eaqbodster.co.uk/Home.html

Hampshire Riding Therapy Centre, Hampshire

A charity committed to working with and educating adults and children with a range of disabilities and special needs.

hampshire-riding-therapy-centre.org.uk

Equine Assisted Therapy Centres, UK

Barton Hill Animal Assisted Therapy Centre

Barton Hill
KENTCHURCH
Herefordshire

www.equine-animal-assisted-therapy.org.uk

The HEART Centre

The Holistic Horse & Pony Centre
Rydings Farm
Long Reach
OCKHAM
GU23 6PF

www.equine-assisted-therapy.com

Red Horse Foundation

Thrupp
STROUD
GL5 2EF

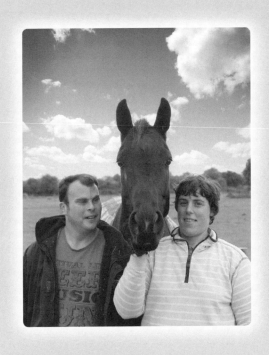

❧ About the author ❧

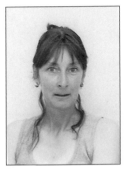Gerry Harrington has previously worked as a registered nurse and certified midwife both in hospitals and in the community. However, her love of horses began when she was a small child and put on the back of a seemingly giant grey horse. With non-horsey parents, the top of her wish list for Christmas and birthdays was always 'A Pony', but she didn't achieve that until she bought her own horse in her late twenties. This boosted her enthusiasm to learn as much as she could about horses, how to care for them and ride with good communication.

After having children of her own and gaining British Horse Society qualifications, she worked at The Fortune Centre of Riding Therapy in the New Forest to mix her nursing and equine careers. She is a great believer in teaching through enjoyment and realised how horses have helped so many people with their problems in life, as just by being near to a horse helps. She went on to gain a degree in teaching and continued working with people with disabilities for many years.

She now supports people to find careers and occupations for themselves in the horse or animal industries and helps provide the opportunity for them to achieve their potential and more self-fulfilment in their lives.